P9-DTV-191

The complete set of books in
Creating Successful Dementia Care Settings
includes

Volume 1: **Understanding the Environment Through Aging Senses**
Volume 2: **Maximizing Cognitive and Functional Abilities**
Volume 3: **Minimizing Disruptive Behaviors**
Volume 4: **Enhancing Identity and Sense of Home**

Training videos for
Creating Successful Dementia Care Settings
include

Maximizing Cognitive and Functional Abilities (companion to Volume 2)
Minimizing Disruptive Behaviors (companion to Volume 3)
Enhancing Self and Sense of Home (companion to Volume 4)
(See ordering information at end of book.)

Creating Successful Dementia Care Settings

Developed by Margaret P. Calkins, M.Arch., Ph.D.

Volume 1
Understanding the Environment Through Aging Senses

Volume Authors
Sherylyn H. Briller, Ph.D.,
Mark A. Proffitt, M.Arch.,
Kristin Perez, OTR/L,
and Margaret P. Calkins, M.Arch., Ph.D.

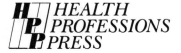
HEALTH
PROFESSIONS
PRESS

Baltimore • London • Winnipeg • Sydney

Health Professions Press, Inc.
Post Office Box 10624
Baltimore, Maryland 21285-0624

www.healthpropress.com

Typeset by Barton Matheson Willse & Worthington, Baltimore, Maryland.
Printed in the United States of America by
The Maple Press Co., York, Pennsylvania.
Interior illustrations by David Fedan.

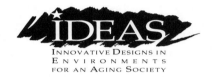

INNOVATIVE DESIGNS IN
ENVIRONMENTS
FOR AN AGING SOCIETY

Margaret P. Calkins, M.Arch., Ph.D., is president of I.D.E.A.S. (Innovative Designs in Environments for an Aging Society), Inc., a consultation, education, and research firm dedicated to exploring the therapeutic potential of the environment as it relates to older adults who are frail and impaired. I.D.E.A.S., Inc., is based in Kirtland, Ohio.

The case examples in this book series are based on the authors' actual experiences. In all instances, names and identifying details have been changed to protect confidentiality.

Library of Congress Cataloging-in-Publication Data

Calkins, Margaret P.
    Creating successful dementia care settings / developed by Margaret P. Calkins.
       p.   cm.
    Includes bibliographical references and index.
    Contents: Vol. 1. Understanding the environment through aging senses—v. 2. Maximizing cognitive and functional abilities—v. 3. Minimizing disruptive behaviors—v. 4. Enhancing identity and sense of home.
    ISBN 1-878812-72-6 (v. 1)—ISBN 1-878812-73-4 (v. 2)—ISBN 1-878812-74-2 (v. 3)—ISBN 1-878812-75-0 (v. 4)
    1. Dementia—Patients—Care. 2. Dementia—Patients—Long-term care. 3. Health facilities—Administration. I. Title.

RC521.C35 2001
362.1'9683—dc21   2001039141

British Cataloguing in Publication Data are available from the British Library.

Series
Contents

Volume 1

Volume 2

Volume 3

Volume 4

About the Authors

Margaret P. Calkins, M.Arch., Ph.D., is President of I.D.E.A.S. Inc. (Innovative Designs in Environments for an Aging Society), a consultation, education, and research firm dedicated to exploring the therapeutic potential of the environment—social and organizational as well as physical—particularly as it relates to older adults who are frail and impaired. She is also Senior Fellow Emeritus of the Institute on Aging and Environment at the University of Wisconsin-Milwaukee.

Dr. Calkins holds degrees in both psychology and architecture. A member of several national organizations and panels that focus on issues of care for older adults with cognitive impairment, she speaks frequently at conferences nationally and internationally. She has published extensively, and her book *Design for Dementia: Planning Environments for the Elderly and the Confused* (National Health Publication, 1998) was the first comprehensive design guide for special care units for people with dementia.

Dr. Calkins is Director and a founding member of SAGE (Society for the Advancement of Gerontological Environments), and has been a juror for numerous design competitions.

Sherylyn H. Briller, Ph.D., is Assistant Professor of Anthropology at Wayne State University. She is a medical anthropologist who specializes in aging research. Dr. Briller received her master's and doctorate degrees and a graduate certificate in gerontology from Case Western Reserve University. She has been actively involved in the field of aging for more than a decade, both domestically and abroad. Her diverse career has included working as an activities coordinator in a skilled nursing facility, a program director at a community senior center, and a gerontological researcher in the United States of America and Asia. Her long-term care expertise includes philosophy/model of care, staff training, activity programming, and ethnic/cultural issues relating to aging. She has consulted, published, and given presentations to numerous audiences including policy makers, researchers, administrators, direct caregivers, and consumers.

John P. Marsden, M.Arch., Ph.D., is an assistant professor in the College of Design, Construction and Planning and a core faculty member of the Institute on Aging at the University of Florida. He holds degrees in architecture from Carnegie Mellon University, the University of Arizona, and the University of Michigan. Dr. Marsden has worked for several architecture firms, was an associate at I.D.E.A.S., Inc., and has consulted with designers and long-term care administrators. He is a frequent speaker at gerontology and environmental design conferences and served as a juror for the 1999 Best of Seniors' Housing Awards, sponsored by the National Council on Seniors' Housing, a division of the National Association of Home Builders.

Kristin Perez, OTR/L, received her bachelor's degree in gerontology from Bowling Green State University and a certificate in occupational therapy from Cleveland State University. Ms. Perez has experience in direct care, programming, management, and research in dementia care settings. She has assisted older adults in maximizing their level of independence and life satisfaction in assisted living, nursing facility, adult day services, and hospital settings. Ms. Perez has been actively involved in numerous research projects addressing dementia care practices and environments, including project management. She has also provided consultation to long-term care facilities regarding dementia care practices and environmental influences.

Mark A. Proffitt, M.Arch., is an architectural researcher with Dorsky Hodgson + Partners, an architectural firm that specializes in designs for older adults. His primary responsibilities include post-occupancy evaluations of completed projects and the programming protocol for the elderly design studio. He strongly believes that good design must build on research. Mr. Proffitt received his master's degree in architecture from the University of Wisconsin–Milwaukee, where he was a fellow with the Institute on Aging and Environment. After receiving his degree, he served as a facilities architect and manager for a developer of retirement communities. Mr. Proffitt has also co-authored a book on the creation and evaluation of an innovative health center and has spoken at several industry-related conferences.

Acknowledgments

Creative endeavors are nurtured to fruition by the ideas and efforts of myriad people at every step of a process. While the original conceptualization for the project was spearheaded by Maggie Calkins, with input from Jerry Weisman, this was very much a team project. All of the authors' talents and contributions were integral and critical to the evolution of the larger project from which these volumes are drawn. In addition, Eileen Lipstreuer, Chari Weber, and Rebecca Meehan deserve as much credit for their contributions to the project as the names that appear on the title pages of these volumes. The videos that accompany these volumes are a direct result of their industriousness. Thanks also to Jesse Epstein, of Cinecraft, and David Litz, the videographer, and to David Fedan for his charming illustrations.

Much of the project was funded by the National Institute on Aging (grant R44 AG12311) and enthusiastically supported and championed by Marcia Ory. We were also fortunate to have a team of nationally recognized experts whose input—both conceptual and practical—was invaluable. We extend our gratitude to Powell Lawton, Jerry Weisman, Phil Sloane, Joe Foley, Susan Gilster, Kitty Buckwalter, Jeanne Teresi, Doug Holmes, and Sheryl Zimmerman. Peter Whitehouse, Elisabeth Koss, Clive Gilmore, and Monte Levinson shared their keen intellect and significant insight with us as we started this project. During the most stressful periods of the project, Cassie and Ted always seemed to come to our rescue.

We would like to thank the numerous individuals whose publications and conference presentations enriched our understanding of the complex nature of dementia, and provided myriad ideas for creative solutions to difficult challenges. We also appreciate the endless hours of listening and thoughtful contributions of the many family, friends, and colleagues who helped out in so many ways as the project evolved over 4 years. To the numerous facility staff and administrators who listened to, read, questioned, and critiqued our efforts and dialogued with us about them, it was for you that we embarked on this voyage. We are pleased to share what we have learned with you.

Preface

All too often, we see well-intentioned caregivers unnecessarily limit or downplay the potential remaining abilities of the older adults with dementia for whom they care. Caregivers seem to assume that because a person has dementia, every behavior and every expression of anxiety, fear, or anger is a direct consequence of the dementing illness. And, because dementia impairs care recipients' cognitive abilities, many caregivers believe that they have the right and the responsibility to make all decisions for those they care for.

It has been the authors' experience that the factors that affect the behavior of residents with dementia are complex. Our approach to understanding their behavior focuses on the person, on his or her typical needs and desires, on the limitations imposed by age-related changes, and on the effects of aspects of the environment.

Our fundamental philosophy is that we must first consider those in our care as people, who have many of the same needs, desires, and wishes as anyone else. To lose the ability to make decisions that affect virtually every aspect of living is devastating. To have that ability further eroded by care providers and care settings that eliminate almost every opportunity for choice and control is unacceptable.

It is the authors' hope that in using the information contained within *Creating Successful Dementia Care Settings*, facilities will create meaningful care settings by educating and sensitizing staff and by making full use of the environmental resources available to them.

User's Guide

The authors' goal in writing this four-volume series was to create an easy-to-use reference to help care providers understand and more appropriately manage, through the environment, the broad array of behaviors and changing abilities that occur with dementia. One must first recognize the importance of accommodating the basic needs of all people, and then one must consider that most people with dementia are older and, therefore, experience the world through sensory modalities that are changing or that have been altered by aging. Vision, hearing, touch, taste, and smell all change with age, and sensory changes often affect behavior. For example, it may not be dementia but simply poor vision that hinders a person's ability to read signs or an activity calendar. Volume 1, *Understanding the Environment Through Aging Senses* helps caregivers to be more sensitive to how these sensory changes can affect a person's basic functioning.

Only after the needs of the resident as a person like anyone else and as an older person with changing sensory experiences have been acknowledged can one consider the unique needs of the individual as an older person with dementia. There is no denying that the neuropathological changes that occur in the brain of a person with dementia affect his or her ability to perceive, make sense of, and operate effectively in the surrounding environment. Basic tasks, such as dressing and eating, that once were easy become increasingly difficult. The inability to interpret what someone is saying, to identify faces or objects, or to understand his or her current location can easily lead to fear and resistance to care. Volumes 2 and 3, *Maximizing Cognitive and Functional Abilities* and *Minimizing Disruptive Behaviors*, respectively, focus on these issues.

Enhancing Identity and Sense of Home, Volume 4, addresses issues that are primarily related to basic human needs such as privacy, autonomy, identity, and personal space. Much of the information is appropriate not only for people with dementia but also for cognitively alert individuals in long-term care settings.

The more that you, as a caregiver, understand all of the factors that affect the person or people whose care is entrusted to you, the better able you are to see the world as they do. Thus, the beginning of each chapter in all of the volumes presents the individual topic from the residents' perspective, including contributing factors and influences on specific behaviors or issues. In addition, these sections offer ideas for assessing problems and implementing interventions. This level of information is particularly useful for staff members who manage and/or train direct care staff. The authors hope that this information will broaden staff's knowledge on the topic and that they will pass the information along to others who care for residents.

The residents' perspective section is followed by "What Staff Can Do," which provides information on social interactions between staff and residents and ideas for structured and spontaneous activities on the unit. Some interventions focus on teaching direct care staff to take a different approach to particular situations, whereas other interventions are provided for staff who plan structured activities and programs.

The third main section of each chapter, "What the Environment Can Do," offers suggestions for modifications or changes that can be made to the physical environment so that your facility becomes more supportive of the residents, particularly those with dementia. Many of the suggested changes cost nothing and involve only a different use of the environment or a small modification using materials you probably already have on hand. Other changes are low in cost, requiring the purchase of a few additional products or materials. Finally, if your facility is able to upgrade or replace some of its furnishings or equipment, we have provided practical advice in "What the Environment Can Do" on what to consider when purchasing a product. Many of the modifications suggested in this section explain how these modifications benefit the residents and the staff who care for them.

The final section of each chapter, "Where to Find Products," lists specific manufacturers and distributors of the products mentioned in the text. There is some repetition in these sections across the four volumes so that you do not have to refer to a separate volume for the information. Many of the manufacturers and catalogs also carry more products than those highlighted in our lists. This section is followed by a summary sheet, which boils down the chapter text into an easy-to-remember, quick overview. We have also provided an area for you to make notes about your own staff and facility. Managerial staff may wish to use the summary sheets as handouts to accompany direct care staff training, or to post them by the time clock or nurses' station or include them in staff's pay envelopes. All staff, including business office, social services, dietary, and housekeeping, may appreciate this quick overview of issues because they likely interact with residents daily.

At the conclusion of each volume, a detailed bibliography and suggested readings help you learn more about issues in the individual volumes. The Behavior Tracking Form and Sensory Stimulation Assessment appendixes appear at the end of Volume 3. Staff can use these forms to examine the occurrence of behaviors and aspects of the environment more closely. Each blank form is accompanied by explanatory information and a sample completed form. Volume 4 includes three appendixes, all designed to help residents feel more at home in the facility and to protect their safety.

In addition to the four volumes, there are three videotapes that relate to Volumes 2–4. They were designed to be staff education resources and provide an additional way of helping all staff learn how to create successful dementia care settings (see ordering information at the end of each volume).

We at I.D.E.A.S., Inc., wish you success in developing a high-quality environment for caregiving. It is our hope that facilities will use this information to create meaningful dementia care settings by educating and sensitizing staff. If you are having a hard time determining which aspects of your care setting most need to be changed or modified, we hope that you will contact us directly (440-256-1880 or info@IDEASconsultingInc.com).

1

The Senses

The five senses—sight, hearing, smell, taste, and touch—provide important biological and social signals that enable us to interpret our world. Although these signals are vital for maintaining physical health, the senses do much more. When you take a walk in a garden, your senses enable you to see the landscape, hear the birds, smell the flowers, and touch the grass. Sensory experiences are a large part of what makes life enjoyable. Sensory stimuli provide several types of information that are vital for well-being. First, they issue warnings about potentially harmful or even life-threatening situations. Second, these signals communicate infor-

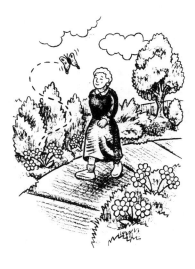

mation that helps people to understand and interpret the environment. Third, these physical signs tell people how to respond appropriately in a given situation and how to react to what they are feeling.

In general, sensory losses occur gradually. People vary as to the rate at which they develop age-related sensory deficits. Some older adults may deny the onset of these physical changes out of vanity, fear, or a belief that nothing can be done because these sensory losses are simply a normal part of aging. Yet, with advancing age, the number of receptor cells and nerve fibers that send sensory stimuli to the brain usually decrease. Therefore, these signals must be stronger for older adults to perceive them (e.g., sounds must be louder, smells must be more intense). Sensory losses can make it difficult for older adults to perform their activities of daily living because most of these activities require the use of multiple senses together.

Sensory impairments also greatly affect the lifestyles of residents of long-term care facilities. When residents cannot see well, it may be difficult for them to locate their rooms or find the way to an activity program. When they do not hear well, it is harder to converse meaningfully with others. Older adults may have trouble smelling food, and reduced senses of smell and taste may make food less tasty than it was when they were younger. These changes often cause older adults to feel socially isolated or depressed. To understand better how residents with sensory losses may feel, try a few of the following sensitivity exercises:

- Wear glasses with petroleum jelly–coated lenses
- Wear earplugs during a meal in the dining room
- Hold your nose and try tasting food
- Put on lightweight gloves and try to do your usual work for an hour or two

Although sensory losses are problematic for all older people, these deficits have a more significant impact on individuals with cognitive impairments. Lowered sensory perception makes it harder for them to function in their environment.

SENSORY STIMULATION

In the field of long-term care, there are several different philosophies about providing sensory stimulation for residents with dementia. The authors believe that appropriate sensory stimulation greatly benefits these residents. Interesting sights, sounds, textures, smells, and tastes provide ways for residents to continue to experience the world. Sensory stimulation also can improve cognition because it helps residents with dementia to maintain interest in their environment. A number of studies also indicate that appropriate sensory stimulation can help maintain functional abilities, improve memory, and increase verbalization (see, e.g., Witucki & Twibell, 1997).

It was once widely believed that low-stimulation units were best for residents with dementia to live on. Researchers since the 1970s have examined how people receive and interpret stimulation from the environment. Lawton and Nahemow (1973) were among the first researchers to theorize that the environment played an increasingly important role as individual competence declined. They developed the environmental docility hypothesis, which suggests that negative consequences occur when the environment is overstimulating. Hall and Buckwalter (1987) also focused on the diminished ability of people with dementia to cope with environmental stimulation. They developed a model known as the progressively lowered stress threshold (PLST). Their findings showed that when residents are unable to cope with existing levels of stimulation, they cross what Hall and Buckwalter termed a *stress threshold,* which results in displays of challenging behaviors. Yet, environments with low to no stimulation can be boring or depressing for residents, who often have nothing to do (Calkins, 1988). When an environment lacks sensory stimulation, residents' concentration and perception may be diminished. They may even experience visual or auditory hallucinations from misperceiving an environment that provides so few cues. Thus, it can be argued that sensory deprivation can contribute to excess disability in residents with dementia. Long-term care staff should imagine how they would feel living in this type of low-stimulus environment and recognize that residents are likely to feel the same way.

Although much early research focused on the quantity of environmental stimulation and its effects on the people being studied, more recent research also has examined the quality of environmental stimulation. There has been little research about how to provide an environment that is interesting yet not overwhelming for these residents, but this is changing. Calkins (1996) considered this issue in significant detail. In her view, positive-quality environmental stimulation may include the following:

- Access to homelike places (e.g., fireplace, front porch)
- Access to outdoor spaces with pleasant places to sit and things to watch
- Pleasant odors (e.g., food, flowers)
- Attractive art and objects that vary in texture

Because positive-quality environmental stimulation is so important, try to devise meaningful activities that are full of sensory cues. When new residents move into your facility, find out from family members what their loved ones' hobbies were (e.g., cooking, gardening) and try to incorporate these activities into their daily routine. There are also many excellent resources that provide suggestions for activities that promote different types of sensory stimulation (e.g., Bowlby, 1993; Nissenboim & Vroman, 1998).

It is also important to recognize that more than just the quantity and quality of stimulation affects people. Too often, long-term care facility environments are filled with conflicting sensory stimuli, which make it hard for residents to move toward positive stimuli while avoiding negative or offensive stimuli. An example is soothing music being played in a living room while a resident is screaming in a nearby tub room; residents with dementia may have trouble screening out the unpleasant background noise and focusing on enjoying the music. Staff should learn how to regulate the levels of sensory stimulation on the dementia-specific unit and provide a variety of positive therapeutic stimuli.

The preceding text has briefly touched on how positive sensory experiences can add to the quality of life of residents with dementia. This discussion is expanded in the following chapters for each of the five senses. Each chapter considers the following aspects:

- Residents' perspectives
- What staff can do
- What the environment can do

2
Vision

Vision provides important sensory cues that residents use in navigating their environment. Too often, older people accept vision impairments because they assume that nothing can be done and that this is a part of normal aging. Yet, most eye conditions can be treated with prescription glasses, contact lenses, medicine, or surgery.

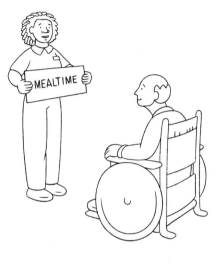

HOW VISION CHANGES WITH AGE

As people age, they experience changes in the eye itself that affect their vision. The size of the pupil decreases, limiting the amount of light that can enter the eye. This means that there must be an increase in the level of light that an object emits or reflects for an older person to see it. The pupil also does not react as quickly to shifts in light levels (e.g., older eyes adjust more slowly when a person comes indoors from a sunny courtyard). A loss of elasticity in the lens of the eye makes it more difficult to change focus between distant and near objects. For this reason, many people in middle age need to wear reading glasses. The lens of the eye also becomes more opaque, which scatters the light entering it and decreases the light intensity that a person can tolerate without experiencing glare. Thickening and yellowing of the lens over time also constrict remaining vision.

Low vision in older adults often is caused by several common eye diseases, including cataracts, diabetic retinopathy, glaucoma, and macular degeneration (Table 2.1). A *cataract* is a clouding of the lens of the eye, which, in general, can be corrected by surgery. More than half of all Americans ages

Table 2.1. Common age-related eye diseases

Disease	Definition
Cataracts	Clouding of the eye's lens causing overall hazy vision
Diabetic retinopathy	Complication of diabetes that damages the retina
Glaucoma	A leading cause of blindness due to excessive intraocular pressure
Macular degeneration	Loss of central vision caused by thinning of the macula (a central region of the retina)

65 and older have cataracts. *Diabetic retinopathy* is a complication of diabetes that affects the retina and can lead to blindness. Approximately half of the 14 million Americans with diabetes have this eye condition, which can be treated with laser surgery or a conventional eye operation. *Glaucoma* results from excessive intraocular (inside the eye) pressure and is one of the leading causes of blindness in older people. The most common form of treatment is medication that reduces this pressure. *Macular degeneration,* the loss of central vision, is another leading cause of blindness in older people. The macula is a small, highly sensitive central region of the retina that allows us to see details and colors well. With aging, this area may become thin and develop yellow spots, and abnormal blood cells may form under it. According to Brawley (1997), there are three types of functional vision losses from these eye diseases of which designers of long-term care facilities should be aware: 1) overall blurred vision, 2) loss of central vision, and 3) loss of peripheral (side) vision.

Overall blurred vision can result from cataracts, corneal scars, or diabetes. Older people with these conditions experience blurred images and heightened sensitivity to glare that results in overall hazy vision. Residents with blurred vision may have trouble seeing well when outside. Because it may be difficult for residents to recognize faces, staff always should identify themselves when approaching residents. This is even more critical when these residents also have dementia.

Loss of central vision is mainly the result of macular degeneration. In older adults with this problem, the central field of vision is affected most and peripheral vision is affected less. Increased light sensitivity and trouble judging colors and recognizing individual features also commonly are associated with this condition. For example, residents may be able to see a staff member approaching but not be able to read his or her name tag.

The loss of peripheral vision results most frequently from either glaucoma or a stroke. With this type of vision loss, people can see only what is directly in front of them. Because they need to turn their heads fully to see things on either side, staff must give careful thought to the placement of furniture in residents' rooms.

Residents with dementia frequently have visual problems that are related to the dementing illness rather than to the aging process. These problems include impaired depth perception, spatial disorientation, altered color perception, and a reduced ability to perceive contrast (Figure 2.1). Some research also suggests that people with dementia take in less visual information. As a result, it is stressful for residents to negotiate their environment when they both do not see well and easily become disoriented. Imagine how upsetting and frightening it is for individuals who see only pieces or parts of things.

Benefits of Natural Lighting

Natural light can do more than increase residents' ability to see well. Too often, residents have little exposure to natural light (i.e., sunlight), which can be beneficial for their health in a number of ways. Beyond helping to synthesize vitamin D through the skin, sunlight also affects the neuroendocrine system. People who are deprived of natural light may suffer from sleep disorders and depression. Inadequate light also has an impact on calcium metabolism, which can contribute to reduced bone mass and osteoporosis (Brawley, 1997).

Low exposure to natural light may negatively affect circadian rhythms. These daily 24-hour cycles influence many biological processes, including body temperature, hormone release, heart rate, blood pressure, and sleep schedules. These rhythms are what cause us to wake up, become hungry, and go to sleep at similar times each day. Alzheimer's disease is sometimes characterized as a rhythmic disorder in which these chemical processes no longer operate properly. Researchers in the field of dementia are studying the relationship of circadian rhythms to bodily function. Some results indicate that conditions that are related to circadian rhythms, such as sleep disorders, seasonal affective disorder, and depression, may occur less frequently if residents of long-term care facilities are exposed to adequate natural light. Using bright light may help reset these biological rhythms.

Another light-related phenomenon with which many nursing facility staff are familiar is sundowning syndrome. In general, this condition occurs in the late afternoon or early evening hours (but can occur in the morning) and results in disruptive and unusual behaviors. The causes are not well understood, but possible explanations include biochemical factors, sensory overload or deprivation, and psychosocial feelings of stress, isolation, or fear. Dehydration, sensory deficits, and low environmental light levels are thought to accentuate sundowning. Thus, turning on lights before dark or using photosensitive lights may help to minimize the occurrence of this behavior at sunset (Evans, 1991).

A

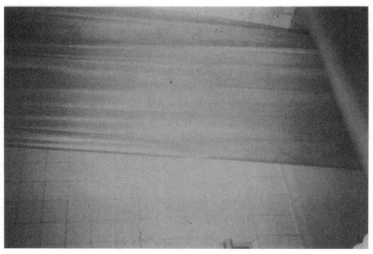

B

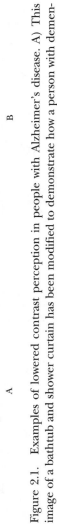

Figure 2.1. Examples of lowered contrast perception in people with Alzheimer's disease. A) This image of a bathtub and shower curtain has been modified to demonstrate how a person with dementia perceives them. B) The same image as seen by a person with normal contrast perception. (Computer simulation of the vision of people with Alzheimer's disease was created with a program developed by Cecil W. Thomas and Grover C. Gilmore of Case Western Reserve University, Cleveland.)

Thus, the environment must be modified to help compensate for some of the visual deficits that are commonly experienced by these residents.

WHAT STAFF CAN DO

Staff should take a proactive approach to enhancing residents' use of their remaining vision. Having up-to-date information about a resident's vision is important in developing an appropriate care plan. In each resident's chart, staff should list types of vision problems and medications/glasses prescribed and document ideas about possible environmental modifications (e.g., rearrangement of the furniture in the bedroom). Staff should periodically review and update the information in this section of the chart.

Staff also should observe how well residents are navigating their environment: Notice whether they are walking into things repeatedly and watch for bruises on their limbs caused by bumping into objects. Should you notice that they are exhibiting unusual behaviors such as pouring salt instead of sugar into their coffee, do not assume that this is a cognitive problem; instead check whether it is related to their vision. Because people with dementia often have impaired verbal communication ability, do not assume that they will tell you about changes in their vision.

Staff should be creative in thinking about ways to increase the functional abilities of residents with low vision. Whether this involves rearranging the furniture in their room, adding new lighting, or using oversized products (e.g., large clocks and signs), these changes can result in significant savings of staff time. Even more important, providing this type of individualized care can make a large difference in residents' overall quality of life.

Before Personal Care

Before administering any personal care, staff always should introduce themselves to residents with dementia, especially those who do not see well. When residents do not know who is speaking to them, they can become intensely frustrated and disoriented. When staff approach a resident to provide personal care, they should explain who they are, what they are going to do, and why they are going to do it. They should use simple language and answer the resident's questions before starting. Doing so greatly reduces the likelihood of combative behavior during personal care. It is well worth taking the extra time to reassure the resident to prevent a catastrophic reaction from occurring.

Keeping Residents Active

When residents do not see well, they may become embarrassed or too fearful to go places and may withdraw socially. Staff can help residents continue to be active by helping them get to activities. Do not assume that residents are able to read activity calendars. Always let them know what is going on each day. When a resident does not attend his or her favorite activity, find out whether the person can find the room in which the activity is held. When a resident stops participating in an activity that he or she used to enjoy, try to figure out the reason why. For example, if the activity is a craft, then maybe the resident is having trouble seeing the beads being used in the activity. Make adjustments for the person, such as using larger beads with bigger holes or providing a place mat in a contrasting color on which to work so that he or she can continue to participate.

> Maria is a very social lady with early-stage Alzheimer disease. She enjoys going to activity programs but has trouble reading the monthly calendar because "the print is too small." Maria also has significant hearing loss and has trouble understanding the overhead announcements giving the time and location of activities. Staff recently noticed that Maria has stopped coming to some of her favorite programs because she cannot remember what day of the week they occur or hear when they are being announced on the public address system. When staff brainstormed, they came up with several ideas to get Maria reinvolved:
> - They made Maria a larger copy of the activity calendar with her favorite programs highlighted.
> - They gave her a magnifying glass to use when reading.
> - A volunteer was assigned to ask Maria whether she wanted to go to her favorite program and help her to find the day room because she has trouble reading the signs.
> - Staff checked Maria's hearing aid battery and reminded Maria to wear her glasses when she went to activities.

Maria soon returned to being highly active after these changes were made.

Staff need to be creative in thinking of ways to help people continue to do the activities that they have enjoyed throughout their lives. Many types of activities, such as music, do not necessarily require sight. For a high-functioning resident with dementia who likes reading, staff can provide large-print books or talking books with earphones; for a low-functioning resident, staff can offer large "coffee table" books filled with colorful pictures. Staff can devise activities that involve more than one sensory experience so that residents with limited vision can participate in the program. For example, a person with low vision can mix dough during a baking activity even if he or she cannot see well enough to measure the ingredients.

WHAT THE ENVIRONMENT CAN DO

Lighting[1]

Lighting is a vital part of every environment because it has a significant impact on what people perceive and do not perceive. There are numerous types of lighting; this section focuses on ambient, indirect, cove, direct, recessed down, task, pendant, and sconce lighting.

Ambient lighting is a uniform system of lighting that is used to brighten an entire space. Ideally, indirect, non–glare-reflecting fixtures should be used so that the interior has even illumination. General ambient lighting should be supplemented by other sources of illumination to provide visual contrast within the environment (Baucom, 1996).

Indirect lighting is a type of ambient lighting in which 90%–100% of the light output is directed toward the ceiling and upper walls (Figure 2.2). In effect, the walls and ceiling become a light source by reflection. When the ceiling color is white or light in tone, the bright surface is perceived visually as receding, and the room appears larger. This illusion can improve visual orientation within larger spaces. It defines the perimeter boundaries when brighter directional lighting is focused on colored vertical surfaces. Overall room illu-

---

[1] Much of the information presented in the definitions in this section was adapted from *Hospitality Design for the Graying Generation: Meeting the Needs of a Growing Market,* by Alfred H. Baucom (New York: John Wiley & Sons, 1996).

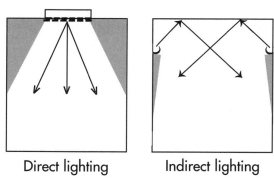

Direct lighting   Indirect lighting

Figure 2.2.   Direct versus indirect lighting.

mination with indirect lighting alone is diffused and shadowless. It can provide a quiet, cool ambiance. One side effect of fully diffused lighting is that it causes a loss of visual contrast and vertical surface texture rendering. Typically, indirect lighting is achieved by using cove lighting, wall sconces, or torchiere floor lamps (floor lamps that project light toward the ceiling; Baucom, 1996).

Cove lighting is a method of indirect lighting in which the light source is attached to the wall and is directed up to a reflective surface. Cove lights should be spaced uniformly to provide even illumination on the ceiling surface because they are used to reflect light from the ceiling to the floor. Used alone, cove lighting can provide general diffused illumination as light is scattered from the reflective ceiling surface (Baucom, 1996).

Direct lighting is light that is directed downward, with the ceiling receiving only the light that is reflected from the floor and furnishings (Figure 2.2). *Direct down lighting* without secondary light sources, such as table lamps, produces shadows on the floor that can confuse older adults. When the ceiling appears dark because of low levels of light that reflect up from the floor and furnishings, the ceiling light sources should be designed with a shielding device such as baffles (or plastic lenses). Shielding devices help reduce glare caused by extreme contrasts in brightness between the dark ceiling and the bright light source (Baucom, 1996).

Recessed-down lighting is a form of direct lighting in which the light source is recessed into a cylinder that is placed above the ceiling. These fixtures focus all of the light downward into a relatively small spot. The beam spread of these fixtures is fairly limited. To be an effective light source, these fixtures must be spaced together tightly to create an even lighting level. Unless these fixtures are located in a high ceiling, the light rarely has a uniform appearance. These fixtures also can create unflattering shadows on people's faces and intense hot spots (bright patches of light that look like a spotlight). Recessed-down lighting is best used as task lighting or to highlight special elements (e.g., art on the wall) rather than as general ambient lighting.

Task lighting is considered a form of direct lighting because light is aimed specifically at an area that the viewer needs to see clearly to accomplish a visual task (e.g., reading). The best task lighting is delivered at angles to improve the contrast between the objects being viewed, such as printed text, and their background. The best visual contrast for reading or writing occurs when light is directed to a task area, such as a tabletop, at angles of approximately 27°, measured vertically from the horizontal surface. Distracting shadows can be reduced when lighting sources are located at both sides of the person performing the task rather than directed at the front and rear of the person (Baucom, 1996).

Pendant lighting is lighting that is hung from the ceiling, such as a chandelier. Pendants can provide direct or indirect lighting or both. Direct lighting from a pendant forces light downward and permits no light to be directed at the ceiling. Indirect pendants force light upward onto only the ceiling surface. Direct/indirect pendants allow light to be directed onto the ceiling and the floor with varying degrees of intensity depending on the fixture. Pendant lighting in long-term care facilities is more effective where the ceilings are higher than 8 feet.

Wall sconces are lighting fixtures that are attached to walls. These fixtures can take several forms and provide either direct lighting or predominantly indirect lighting. Similar to pendants, indirect wall sconces reflect most of the available light onto the walls and ceiling, whereas direct wall sconces reflect light downward or outward. Combinations of both types are possible. Wall sconces must be used as a secondary, rather than a primary, ambient light source because, in general, they do not generate enough light to illuminate an entire room.

Color rendering refers to the ability of a light source to render colors that are as close to daylight as possible. All colors look different when viewed in varying forms of light. Colors should look like they are being viewed in daylight conditions. However, even daylight is seen in varying degrees of light, so "daylight" is an arbitrary condition within a defined range of light. The Color Rendering Index for lamps uses 100 as the number for light that most closely resembles typical daylight. Any bulb with a number of 80 or higher indicates a reasonably accurate color rendering (Baucom, 1996).

Another measure of color rendering is degrees Kelvin (° K), a measure of the color of a black object while burning. At different temperatures the black object glows in varying colors of light. (An analogy is noticing how the flame in a campfire is hotter where it glows blue rather than orange.) Incandescent lights are rated at 3000° K. There are multiple types of fluorescent bulbs with ratings between 2700° and 3500° K. These bulbs are referred to as *daylight, cool white, warm white, cool white deluxe, and warm white deluxe.* The cool white bulb is the least expensive but has the worst color rendering. Bulbs with better color rendering and appearance are the cool white deluxe, daylight, and warm white deluxe. The recommended light ratings that simulate either daylight conditions or incandescent lighting are 3000°–3500° K.

Ways to Improve Poor or Inadequate Lighting

Finding a balance between noninstitutional-looking and functional lighting can be challenging. The section "How People Change Physically with Age" described some of the negative biological effects that may occur when the lighting in long-term care facilities is inadequate. Because residents with dementia are less likely than those without dementia to make adjustments that would help them to see better (e.g., staying away from glare, turning on additional lights), it is critical for facilities to have in place good-quality lighting systems to maximize residents' functioning.

Lighting Levels

Proper illumination is often based on the appropriate placement of light. Proper illumination both brightens the visual environment and enhances the functional abilities of residents with limited vision. It also increases safety and helps residents with poor vision to navigate their environment more easily. Because a 60-year-old person needs two to three times more light than does a 20-year-old to perform the same task (Brawley, 1997), staff may not be the most accurate judge of the adequacy of the light level for residents. Several steps can be taken to assess the amount of light that is needed by residents. A simple first step in determining whether the facility has adequate light is for staff members to wear a pair of sunglasses inside for several hours. Attention should be paid to how well they can recognize faces, read signs, and see across a room. If this exercise causes staff to believe that the facility may not be lit properly, then a more accurate measure of the light levels should be obtained.

A common measure of light level is the footcandle, which measures the amount of light in a room. Footcandle meters can be purchased at some camera and school supply stores to test the environment. (If the light meter reads in lux, then divide the number by 100, which results in the footcandle measurement.) Hold the light meter about 2½ feet from the floor when taking readings. Use the levels in Table 2.2 to determine whether minimal lighting

Table 2.2. Minimum ambient light levels

Activity areas (day only)	30 footcandles
Living room (day)	30 footcandles
Barber/beautician (day)	50 footcandles
Chapel or quiet area (active)	30 footcandles
Hallways (active hours)	30 footcandles
Hallways (sleeping hours)	10 footcandles
Dining (active hours)	50 footcandles
Interior entry (day)	100 footcandles
Interior entry (night)	10 footcandles
Exit stairway/landings	30 footcandles
Elevator interiors	30 footcandles
Physical therapy area (active hours)	30 footcandles
Occupational therapy (active hours)	30 footcandles
Resident's room	30 footcandles
Wardrobe	30 footcandles
Bathroom entry	30 footcandles
Bathroom	30 footcandles
Make-up/shaving area	30 footcandles
Shower/bathing rooms	30 footcandles

From Illuminating Engineering Society of North America. (1998). *Recommended Practice for Lighting and the Visual Environment for Senior Living.* Document No. RP-28-98. New York: Author.

levels are being met. This table is based on the Illuminating Engineering Society of North America's schedule for light levels, and the levels are calculated based on the age of the user. However, the guidelines provided cover only the eyesight of people at about age 50. There is no accurate study of the light levels that are required for people in their 70s and 80s. Therefore, these numbers should be used only as minimums, and facilities should consider implementing higher light levels. Significant variations in light levels within a room by 25 footcandles or more indicate that there is room for improvement. Another rule of thumb is to take the lowest reading in the room and multiply it by 3. No reading in the room should be higher than the resulting number.

It is important for facilities to provide even and consistent lighting to avoid confusing or frightening shadows. Keep in mind, however, that some shadows are necessary to help residents understand their environment. Because the ability to discern edges is diminished in people with Alzheimer's disease, it is important to provide some direct light to create shadows that help to visually define edges in rooms where residents perform tasks. Many long-term care facilities have begun to use indirect lighting systems such as indirect pendant and cove lighting to create higher levels of even ambient illumination. However, the exclusive use of indirect light provides very flat lighting. Shadows that define the edges of items are less visible in indirect light. Light from other sources should be added through the use of table and floor lamps.

Staff need to make informed decisions about improving lighting. Shop around for an interior designer or a lighting sales representative who provides a full range of services. One important service is a footcandle plot. A footcandle plot shows the light level of the room based on the ceiling height, type of fixtures, and spacing of the light fixtures. The light level should meet minimum ambient light levels (see Table 2.2), and it should be fairly consistent. Again, the numbers on the plot should not fluctuate more than 25 footcandles in the room. If a footcandle plot is not available, then consider testing the proposed lighting scheme in one room first by comparing light levels against the numbers that are provided in Table 2.2.

Focused Task Lighting

Carefully examine the lighting in the areas where residents perform tasks for which good vision is required. Additional lighting can help maximize residents' abilities to complete focused tasks such as dressing or grooming. Brighter lighting not only helps residents with dementia to see better but it also may help them to concentrate on the task (see Table 2.3). Standard task lighting usually comes from table or floor lamps. Make sure that the lamps that are selected do not produce intense glare. Halogen bulbs are useful because they provide bright, intense light for tasks. They also can become extremely hot, however, so it is important to keep the bulbs out of residents' reach. If lamps are within easy reach of residents, then use compact fluorescent bulbs, which are cooler to the touch.

Bulbs and Ballasts

Proper bulb and ballast selections can make a difference in improving lighting. Without changing any fixtures, a facility can dramatically improve the quality of its lighting by installing the proper bulbs. Use bulbs that provide good color rendering, so colors appear true. Improper bulbs can make skin tones look

Table 2.3.   Minimum task light levels

Make-up/shaving area	60 footcandles
Closet	75 footcandles
Reading chair	50–100 footcandles
Shower/bathing	50 footcandles

jaundiced or make food look unappetizing. When replacing existing or installing new fluorescent bulbs, use full-spectrum bulbs. These bulbs have high color rendering and reduce eye fatigue. An alternative to full-spectrum bulbs is to mix different fluorescent bulbs such as warm white deluxe and cool white deluxe. Any bulb with a Color Rendering Index of 80 or higher or a rating of 3000°–3500° K also provides reasonable color rendering.

The national energy code (ASHRAE/IESNA 90.1-1999) specifies using fluorescent bulbs for general lighting in most care settings to reduce energy consumption. Using incandescent bulbs instead can provide a warm, cozy atmosphere, which may be more appropriate in some areas of the facility. Although incandescent lights can make a room appear warmer, these lights emphasize yellow tones, which already may be heightened by older vision. Thus, incandescent bulbs are not recommended as a primary light source but rather as an accent to a general lighting scheme. Some incandescent bulbs are full spectrum to portray colors accurately, so facilities should spend the extra money for these full-spectrum bulbs. Also, use frosted incandescent bulbs to diffuse light and reduce glare.

Fluorescent bulbs dim and flicker after extended use. Flickering can lead to agitation among residents, and dim lights can contribute to falls. Every facility should have a replacement policy to prevent these incidents from occurring. All fixtures should be checked for flickering and dimming bulbs at least once per month. Fluorescent lights have ballasts that convert electrical energy into light. When replacing existing or installing new ballasts, use an electronic ballast, which reduces the flickering and the hum that is associated with a magnetic ballast. This hum can be extremely annoying to residents with hearing aids. Dimmers can be installed on fluorescent fixtures with electronic ballasts so that lighting can be adjusted to mimic daylight conditions. The energy efficiency of these ballasts often pays for the replacement costs over time.

If the facility does not have electronic ballasts and/or dimmers, then some of the fixtures can be switched separately. This permits the adjustment of lighting levels to complement daylight conditions in the room and the creation of different ambiances. More information regarding lighting for specific areas is provided in various sections of Volume 2 (e.g., see Chapter 5 for dining room lighting, Chapter 3 for hallway lighting, and Chapter 6 for closet lighting).

Glare

Glare is a source of intense light in a person's immediate view. Glare greatly contributes to excess disability because it reduces attention span, adds to confusion and agitation, and increases the risk of falls. Light sources, both daylight

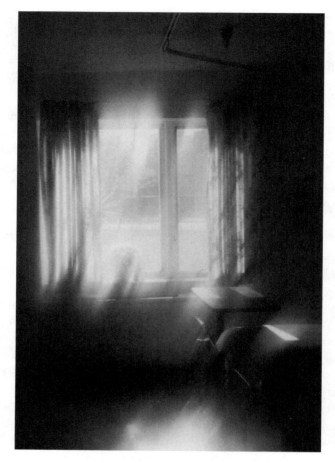

Figure 2.3.   The effect of direct and indirect glare from windows.

and artificial, should be balanced to minimize glare, which makes the environment more comfortable and safer for residents. There are two broad categories of glare. The first type is *direct glare*, which is intense light emanating from an immediate source. Examples include unshielded light bulbs or direct sunlight streaming through windows. The second type is *indirect glare*, which is intense light that is reflected from a surface, such as a shiny floor. Windows and the area around windows often give off both types of glare (Figure 2.3).

Because residents are sensitive to glare, all of the windows in a care setting should have some means of filtering or blocking light. Vertical and horizontal blinds are not the best choice because they create alternating slits of light and darkness that can be disorienting to residents with dementia. When metal blinds are used, the light may reflect off the blinds, causing even more glare. Window treatments in facilities should be sheers or translucent shades, which allow light to be diffused without totally blocking the view. Windows also should be equipped with curtains or opaque shades to cover the window completely. The reason is that, at night, windows can act like mirrors, which can be disturbing to residents. In addition, intense light from western and/or eastern exposures can be problematic for residents.

Shiny, clean floors are a source of indirect glare in health care settings (Calkins, 1988). It is important to know that "clean" does not have to mean "shiny." Instead of polishing floors, consider buffing floors with a cleanser that leaves a matte finish. Administrators may be concerned that some families will be upset by this method because they may think that the facility is not as clean as it was when the floors were shiny. If this is the case, then administrators may want to write letters to the family members of residents to explain that the facility is eliminating shiny floors because the glare from them is detrimental to residents' well-being.

Older adults' eyes adjust slowly to changes in light levels in areas of transition from bright to moderate light (e.g., doorways from the outside). To accommodate these adjustments, the facility should provide places where an older person can sit and rest while his or her eyes adjust. Lighting in the vestibule can be increased during the day and decreased at night. Also, options should be available for adjusting light levels over the course of a day to orient residents to the passage of time. This can be especially helpful in minimizing the effects of sundowning syndrome.

Color and Pattern

Benefits of Color

The topic of color is somewhat controversial among researchers who study dementia, and there is ongoing debate regarding the therapeutic benefits of color. Researchers do not yet fully understand the extent of color perception deficits in people with dementia. It is believed, however, that because the lens of the eye yellows with age, older people do have trouble differentiating between certain colors (e.g., between blues and greens; Brawley, 1997). This research may have an impact on the choice of colors that are used when designing special care units for people with dementia. Some helpful guidelines are to choose colors that older people are able to see well and to use contrasting colors to help them differentiate among aspects of the environment.

Use brighter colors for objects that residents should see (e.g., resident bedroom signs) and muted colors or colors that are similar to those used in the background for objects that residents should not see (e.g., locked exit doors). When the facility has rooms or areas that are habitually cool, they can be made to feel warmer through the use of bright, warm colors (e.g., yellows, reds, oranges). A warm room can be made to feel cooler by using cool colors (e.g., blues, greens). One way to test how the color scheme will appear to residents is to look at the chosen colors through a piece of yellow acetate. The acetate helps to mimic the way that older eyes are likely to perceive these colors. The samples should be viewed in the same light as that in the room in which the colors will be used.

Color contrast helps residents with low vision to distinguish among different types of objects in the environment. Studies have shown that "healthy older persons require about three times as much contrast as younger persons for the detection of objects in the environment" (Tideiksaar, 1997, p. 53). Increasing the contrast between objects (furniture) and the background (walls, floors) helps residents to see better. For example, contrast is improved when a room has a darker wall and a lighter colored floor. The color of features such as tabletops and countertops should contrast with the color of the floors. Adding a contrasting-colored edge is a low-cost way to make this change, which helps residents to differentiate between these surfaces better. Similarly, a brightly colored or black toilet seat with a white bathroom floor is easier for residents to see and can reduce episodes of incontinence.

Pattern

There are pros and cons to using patterns in areas occupied by residents with dementia. Because these residents often have problems with spatial relationships, facilities should consider carefully how different types of patterns might affect residents' ability to see and maneuver in the environment. Some residents may become dizzy or disoriented by large geometric patterns. Wavy or undulating patterns may appear to move and cause residents to experience unsteadiness or they may induce hallucinations. Residents with dementia may also misperceive features such as stripes for bars.

A good use of pattern can help in creating a more homelike feeling in a facility. Most older adults prefer classic patterns that are similar to those that were in their homes, as opposed to contemporary ones. In general, smaller patterns are best, but before you buy specific patterns, consider how they may make residents react. If possible, test new patterns in one area first to see how residents respond to the change. Although some studies have been done comparing the use of patterns in various settings, there are no solid research results suggesting that there is a single correct solution to this issue. For a more elaborate discussion of residential design issues, see Volume 4.

Room Features

Bedrooms

Appropriate signs for bedrooms and personal orientation cues help residents visually recognize their bedrooms. Place signs on the section of the bedroom door where the resident is most likely to see them. For example, if the resident uses a wheelchair or walks stooped over, then the sign should be placed on the bottom half of the door. Lower signage is allowed under ADA guidelines as long as the facility can show that the variation from the ADA–recommended heights are a better accommodation to the residents' individual strengths and limitations. "The goal [of the ADA] is to design environments that support the strengths that people have, and to 'reasonably accommodate' their limitations" (Kearney, 1992, p. 21). Adequate lighting both in and around residents' bedrooms is important so that residents can identify their rooms correctly. If the facility uses special orientation cues to mark bedroom doorways (e.g., display cases filled with personal objects), then these areas must be well lit for residents to see them. (See Volume 2, Chapter 2 for further suggestions about designing good cueing systems.)

Ask families to provide artwork for the residents' rooms— preferably pieces of art from their homes. This increases the likelihood that residents will visually identify with and recognize their rooms. If a certain picture always hung over the dresser at home, then hang it over the dresser in the resident's room. It may help cue him or her as to the purpose of this piece of furniture. Observe residents as to whether they have positive or negative reactions to artwork in their rooms. If a piece of artwork appears to frighten a resident, then remove it; the resident may perceive it differently than do staff because of his or her dementing illness.

Common Areas

Because low vision can make people feel socially isolated, areas where residents often sit and have conversations should be arranged thoughtfully. A lamp placed next to a group of chairs should enable a resident with poor vision to be able to see the faces of others he or she is talking to more easily. Also, chairs should be placed together to form small, intimate groups of residents rather than long rows of people.

Bookcases or shelves with items of interest for the residents to browse among should be paired with lamps or other direct lighting in the area to draw residents' attention and make it easier for them to see what is available. Oversized accessories such as clocks and calendars with large numbers and telephones with large buttons maximize the functional abilities of residents with low vision. Make sure that there is bright, even lighting in the social spaces. Also, try to reduce glare by carefully considering both the placement of furniture and the use of window treatments. For instance, the television should be placed so that glare from the windows is not reflected on the screen.

◆ ◆ ◆

A summary sheet follows, which condenses the chapter text into a quick overview. The authors have also provided an area for you to make your own notes about your own staff and facility. Managerial staff may wish to use the summary sheets as handouts to accompany direct care staff training, or to post them by the time clock or nurses' station or include them in staff's pay envelopes.

VISION SUMMARY SHEET

Vision provides sensory cues that help people navigate the environment. Some visual impairments can be treated with glasses, contact lenses, medication, or surgery. The eye changes in the following ways as people age:

1. The pupil becomes smaller, requiring more light to see clearly. It opens/closes more slowly, making it difficult to adjust when a person moves from a dark to a bright space and vice versa.

2. The lens loses elasticity; the adjustment that must be made from viewing tasks that are done close up to those done at a distance from the eye is more difficult than in a person's youth.

3. The lens becomes more opaque, making it difficult to tolerate glare.

4. The lens thickens and yellows, affecting overall vision.

5. Diseases of the eye such as cataracts, diabetic retinopathy, glaucoma, and macular degeneration may develop or become worse. Blurred vision or loss of central/peripheral/side vision are some of the effects of these diseases.

6. People with dementia experience additional problems with vision in such areas as depth perception, spatial disorientation, and identifying colors/seeing contrasts.

What Staff Can Do

1. Observe how well residents function and get around in the environment. If they get lost easily, bump into things and bruise frequently, or demonstrate odd behaviors such as mistaking salt for sugar, then they may have vision problems.

2. In each resident's records and during caregiver orientation list the type of vision loss and the known visual aids each resident uses (e.g., glasses) increased light, and/or other environmental changes.

3. Try rearranging furniture; adding large-print books, clocks, and signs; introducing yourself by name at the beginning of each interaction with residents who do not see well; encouraging activity and adapting tasks or task materials; testing light levels yourself by wearing sunglasses in the environment to determine whether you can easily read signs, recognize faces, or eat a meal.

What the Environment Can Do

1. Increase overall lighting and task lighting without creating glare.

2. Create evenly lit spaces; note that some shadows at the room's perimeter should be retained.

3. Mix the types of light sources.

4. To avoid glare, cover light bulbs and use shades and sheer curtains in dining rooms, reading rooms, and craft areas.

5. Provide spaces where residents can adjust to changes in light levels (e.g., from room to room); provide low-glare floor surfaces.

6. Use contrasting colors in the environment to help people find light switches, wall edges, and doorways.

7. Properly light and make highly visible all bedroom/bathroom entrances and signs.

8. Use personal items outside and within bedrooms as cues for residents to identify their room and to provide continuity with their past.

9. Ensure adequate lighting to help people read or see others while conversing.

10. Arrange seating, dining tables, and television screens to avoid glare from windows.

YOUR NOTES

3
Hearing

Hearing is one of the first senses that are affected by the normal processes of aging. The National Institutes of Health reported that between one third and two thirds of adults ages 65 and older are hard of hearing (Brawley, 1997). Most age-related hearing losses occur gradually but become more severe with advancing age. Hearing losses often make communication 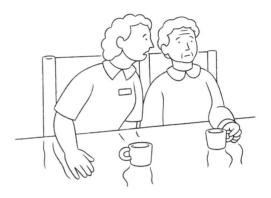 more difficult, causing some older adults to withdraw socially. Many older people simply give up and tell themselves that it does not matter if they cannot hear what others are saying. They may view it as too much work (or too embarrassing) to constantly ask people to repeat themselves.

HOW HEARING CHANGES WITH AGE

Age-related hearing decline (*presbycusis*) is a common problem. With advancing age, the number of nerve cells that conduct sound signals to the brain decreases. There are also changes in the cochlea, an organ in the inner ear that transforms mechanical sound waves into nerve impulses. The region of the cochlea that is most sensitive to high-frequency sounds is affected the most. As early as age 40, many people begin to experience losses in their ability to hear high-frequency pitches. Losing the ability to hear the upper frequencies is similar to listening to a radio that is not tuned clearly to one station. Increasing the volume only makes the background noise seem more obvious and distracting. Thus, when you are speaking to people who are hard of hearing, talking louder does not necessarily help them to hear better (Baucom, 1996).

Older people have more difficulties with speech discrimination and take longer to process auditory information than do younger people. Whereas each sound is a single tone or frequency, speech is a complex set of tones. In general, consonants are harder than vowels to hear because they do not carry as much power. Consonants that have a higher frequency component in their acoustical pattern (s, z, t, f, g) are much more difficult to hear. Background noise tends to mask these weaker speech sounds, making them even harder to comprehend. Because consonants contain much of the information that is conveyed in words, difficulty in hearing consonants may have an adverse effect on an older person's ability to understand the speech of others.

WHAT STAFF CAN DO

Communicating with a resident with a hearing impairment can be challenging. Some residents may not recognize or admit that they have difficulty hearing. They may blame others for mumbling or not speaking clearly. In certain cases, residents may become paranoid and think that others are talking about them all of the time. Not hearing well can result in misunderstandings between residents and staff.

Factors that can affect how well a resident is able to hear include the following:
- The pitch of the speaker's voice
- The direction in which the speaker is facing
- The cognitive processing and attention span of the resident
- The level of background noise

Residents' ability to hear also may vary on different days depending on how they are feeling, the weather and amount of air pressure, and what is going on in the environment (e.g., construction work).

Staff should not assume that because a resident responds inappropriately, the problem is always the result of his or her dementing illness. However, staff should be attentive to whether a resident's hearing is changing over time. In particular, a resident with dementia may not realize that his or her hearing is getting worse or say anything about this to staff. When they do not hear well, residents may
- Have a noncommittal expression on their faces
- Exhibit slow or inappropriate responses
- Tend to lean forward, straining to hear

- Tilt their heads to one side to hear
- Peer into speakers' faces to understand what is being said
- Fail to respond
- Be inattentive
- Be unable to recognize when they are speaking loudly or softly

Communication Techniques

Not being able to hear can be detrimental to the quality of life of older people in many ways. Furthermore, because hearing losses cause excess disability for residents with dementia, it is important to take all possible steps to maximize communication with these residents. Each resident's hearing should be assessed by an audiologist when he or she moves into the facility and at periodic intervals afterward (about once per year). In each resident's chart, staff should list hearing problems and document effective strategies for communicating with the person (e.g., always speak directly into Mrs. Smith's left ear). In addition to keeping this information in the resident's chart (which is required by law), write this information—as well as other important care tips—on an index card for each resident. That way, when new or regular staff work with residents with whom they are less familiar, they can easily put these cards in a pocket for easy reference during their shift and will know what strategies work best for each resident. It is wise to keep multiple copies of these cards in case staff forget to return them at the end of their shift.

Staff should speak to residents with hearing problems while facing them at eye level and should not shout but rather raise their voices slightly. The increased volume during shouting actually heightens the register of the voice, making it more difficult to hear. This accentuates the vowels and masks the consonants that these residents already find difficult to hear. Age-related deficits also commonly affect one ear more than the other. If a resident has a significant hearing loss in the right ear, then approach him or her on the left side and speak directly into the left ear. Be patient and repeat the statement or question slowly if the resident does not hear it the first time, or try saying it another way that he or she may hear or comprehend better.

Staff must be creative and use multiple types of sensory information to communicate with a resident. Supplement what you are saying with visual cues such as facial expressions and gestures to clarify the meaning. If a resident can read, then write notes or use cards with simple graphics to indicate the message (e.g., mealtime, bath time). These materials should be kept simple and should cover only what is essential for the resident to know.

Socialization

Residents with hearing impairment should be given good seats in activity programs where they can hear better as well as see the ongoing events. If these residents become withdrawn and avoid conversing with others, then provide quiet social spaces with little background noise where they can visit one-to-one and have a cup of coffee with one other resident, a family member, or a volunteer. Staff should devise other activities that these residents can enjoy. If their vision is not impaired, then they can be given attractive things to look at, such as colorful magazines or craft projects. Those whose hearing and vision are both poor can be given interesting things to touch, smell, and taste.

WHAT THE ENVIRONMENT CAN DO

The environment can make a major difference in terms of the degree of excess disability experienced by residents who have hearing problems. Poorly designed spaces can magnify their problems, whereas well-designed spaces can help to compensate for some of these deficits. The physical environment should enable residents to maximize the use of their remaining hearing.

Excess Noise

Background noise greatly affects residents with hearing losses. It is particularly disturbing for those who wear hearing aids because most of these devices magnify background noise. When this noise irritates residents with dementia, they can become agitated and restless or may try to leave the unit. The unit should be as quiet and peaceful as possible. The overall noise level on the unit can be lowered in the following ways:

- Do not play background music, such as "canned" music.
- Eliminate loud televisions, radios, and other disturbing noises.
- Avoid calling out or yelling to other staff members.
- Limit the use of the public address system only to emergencies rather than using it for convenience.
- Turn off call bells and alarm systems quickly.
- Lubricate squeaky wheels on carts and wheelchairs.
- Change the scheduling of noisy tasks such as vacuuming to times when residents are not socializing.

Acoustical Treatments for Hard Surfaces

Residents will not hear as well in a room filled with hard surfaces because sound reverberates more when the surfaces of ceiling, walls, and floor all are hard. Many residential facilities have acoustical tile ceilings. However, if the remainder of the surfaces are resilient, sound will reverberate for a long time before the ceiling tile has any absorbent effect. In rooms where large numbers of residents assemble, such as dining and activity rooms, the best solution is to provide for sound absorption on the walls, ceiling, and floors.

In open public spaces, ambient background noise reverberates and should be muffled by using additional materials such as fabric wall hangings or fabric acoustical wall coverings. In areas in which "cleanability" is important, soundproofing panels can be used as an accent wall or to create a decorative pattern on the walls. These panels can be covered with microperforated fabric coverings that can be wiped down with a damp cloth. These coverings are available in a variety of colors and patterns. In wet areas such as tub rooms, Tedlar-covered acoustical panels, which are water resistant, can be used.

Because window glass is a hard surface, drapery, wall, and window treatments should be used to help modify poor acoustic conditions in rooms with many windows. Full drapery treatments have better acoustical benefits than just valances or vinyl blinds. If sound in the room is a significant problem, then lined draperies can be considered as well. Furniture and other movable items that are soft or porous can reduce sound. The backs of chairs frequently are made of a soft breathable fabric that helps to absorb sound. Use vinyl, laminated fabrics, or a product like Scotchguard on the seat, where moisture resistance is important.

The noise-reducing factor in facilities with ceiling tiles should be as high as possible in rooms where people congregate. Ceiling tiles are most effective when they are installed 9 feet above the floor and there is 2½ feet of clearance between the ceiling tiles and the structure of the floor above

(McGuinness, Stein, & Reynolds, 1980). Therefore, if the installation of the ceiling tile is not optimum, existing panels should be replaced with panels of the highest Noise Reduction Criteria (NRC) rating possible. A good panel has a rating of at least 0.75 or higher (the higher the number, the better the rating). If the facility has a drywall ceiling or soffit in the dining room, then an acoustical spray finish can be added to reduce noise.

Studies have shown that background noise can be reduced by 70% when carpeting is added to a room (Baucom, 1996). Because of advances in technology, carpeting can be considered in almost all residential areas (e.g., see Volume 2, Chapter 5 for a comparison of carpeting and resilient flooring).

◆ ◆ ◆

A summary sheet follows, which condenses the chapter text into a quick overview. The authors have also provided an area for you to make your own notes about your own staff and facility. Managerial staff may wish to use the summary sheets as handouts to accompany direct care staff training, or to post them by the time clock or nurses' station or include them in staff's pay envelopes.

HEARING SUMMARY SHEET

1. Age-related hearing loss progresses slowly, but by age 65 from one third to two thirds of adults are hard of hearing.

2. By age 40 many people have lost their ability to hear high-pitched (high frequency) sounds. When people speak, some letters may be harder for older people to hear. Processing sounds and words may take longer. People are often unaware of their own hearing losses.

3. Poor hearing can result in misunderstandings between residents and between residents and staff. Factors that affect hearing negatively include voice pitch, the position of the speaker to the person hearing him or her, cognitive processing and the attention span of the listener, and background noise. Illness also can be a factor. In some facilities, some residents are presumed to have dementia when they actually have impaired hearing.

4. Signs of possible hearing loss can include a noncommittal facial expression, a slow or inappropriate response, leaning forward/straining to hear, always tilting the head to the same side, peering into your face to understand what is being said, a failure to respond, inattentiveness, and/or an inability to recognize whether a person is speaking softly or loudly.

5. Hearing loss affects the quality of life and creates excess disability. It is important to make the most of each resident's ability to communicate.

What Staff Can Do

1. Arrange a professional hearing assessment for residents who you think might have difficulty hearing.

2. Residents' records should document their type of hearing difficulty. All staff who work with a particular resident should be made aware of the best way to approach the person or speak to him or her: In general, approach the "good ear" or face him or her at eye level. Speak clearly and keep the tone or register of the voice low. It may be helpful to raise the volume of the voice, but only slightly. If the staff member is not heard/understood the first time, then he or she should carefully choose words, try to keep statements brief, and repeat them. If the resident has a hard time understanding a particular word, then try restating the sentence using a different word. Staff should provide additional cues by using facial expressions and gestures. They should try using short written notes or pictures.

3. Make sure that residents can hear and see well, especially during activities. Sit near them and interpret if necessary. Provide quiet corners for one-to-one visits and small group discussions. Include activities that offer interesting sights, smells, and tactile experiences.

What the Environment Can Do

1. Background noise is especially difficult for people who have a hearing impairment. It distorts sound, interferes with hearing aids, and disturbs residents with

dementia. Lower the overall noise level by turning off background music. Turn off televisions and radios or shut doors to rooms in which they are playing.

2. Avoid yelling or calling down hallways and quickly turn off call bells. Find quiet alternatives to public address systems or use them only for emergencies. Schedule noisy tasks when they would least affect residents' socializing, and fix squeaky carts or other equipment.

3. Rooms with hard surfaces increase hearing difficulty. Wall hangings, soundproof panels, lined drapes, furniture lined with fabric, acoustic ceiling treatments, and carpeting help to absorb sound.

YOUR NOTES

4

Smell and Taste

Smell and taste are among the most important types of sensory information that residents receive during the day. For instance, the smell of freshly brewing coffee in the morning may cue residents that it is time for breakfast. For those who have awakened to that same smell for most of their lives, this type of familiar experience can be comforting and help to maintain lifelong patterns. As cognitive processes decline with advancing dementia, the senses of smell and taste may become increasingly important sensory cues for these residents.

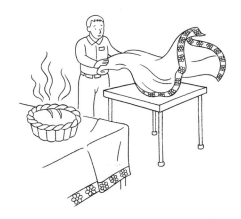

HOW SMELL AND TASTE CHANGE WITH AGE

We often have a strong emotional response to odors because our olfactory sense is integrally linked with our limbic system, the part of the brain that deals with emotion and memory processing. Smell actually reaches the brain more quickly than other senses, such as sight and sound. Whereas pleasant smells may be comforting and relaxing, bad odors can increase stress and affect the breathing and heart rates of residents. Furthermore, they can cause agitation and even lead to catastrophic reactions in some residents. People with dementia appear to have more problems discriminating among smells than do other older adults.

A decrease in the number of taste buds accounts for increasing difficulties with taste after age 50. Typically, there is a lowered ability to discriminate between the four components of taste: sweet, sour, bitter, and salty. Reduced senses of smell and taste also often contribute to a diminished ability to enjoy food, which can lower appetite and contribute to significant weight loss. Residents with dementia commonly experience eating difficulties, and sensory impairments may compound these problems.

WHAT STAFF CAN DO

Incorporating Positive Smells and Tastes

There are many smells that are part of daily life from home that residents may miss. These include the scent of freshly mown grass, cookies baking, or laundry taken fresh from a clothesline. Because smells can influence residents' moods significantly, try to add positive familiar aromas in the environment. Use good smells and tastes in all kinds of activities for residents with dementia. These aromas and tastes can stimulate reminiscence about certain lifelong seasonal patterns, such as baking holiday cookies in the winter or picking fresh herbs from a summer garden. These sensory experiences can help to orient residents with dementia to the time of year.

Incorporate positive smells when providing personal care for residents with dementia to reduce agitation and promote relaxation. For example, fragrant baths can help residents to relax and feel like they are taking a bath at home instead of in an institutional setting. Bubble bath, scented shower gels, shaving cream, even the smell of hairspray may be familiar and comforting and may minimize episodes of agitation during personal care. Some residents may feel calmer if they are given a washcloth with scented soap or a puff with scented powder to use in the bathroom. This technique can be employed at other times besides bathing. For example, residents can be given a handkerchief that is scented with lavender or a favorite perfume or cologne to carry with them throughout the day.

Older people generally prefer more intense flavors because their sense of taste may be diminished. Lemonade for activity programs should be made a little sweeter or coffee a little stronger so that residents can appreciate these familiar flavors.

Using Smells with Personal Meaning

The resident's social history may indicate the smells and tastes to which he or she may personally respond. A mother who raised many children may enjoy having a container of baby powder on her dresser. A former baker may like having a vanilla-scented container to carry around that he can open and enjoy. Also, families should be asked what scents the resident always wore and preferred. Staff should observe whether a resident favors certain scents by looking closely at his or her facial expression. Does the person appear relaxed and content or tearful and upset? The scent may trigger a memory that is painful (e.g., the smell of a certain perfume reminds the resident of his or her mother, making the resident feel lost or lonely). This information should be indicated in the resident's chart so that new staff can learn the resident's likes and dislikes. Document which scents have already been tried to let other staff know the resident's preferences.

Minimizing Negative Smells

Negative institutional smells such as strong cleaning fluids should be replaced with more homelike odors such as a cleanser that is lemon scented. Nontoxic potpourri or floral- or pine-scented air fresheners can add other homelike smells in the facility.

If certain residents frequently have unpleasant body odors, others may not want to socialize with or be near them. This can be damaging psychologically; these residents may feel lonely and depressed. Social isolation and inability to interact with others also can have a negative impact on their cognition. Staff can help by ensuring that residents with unpleasant body odors bathe more frequently and get their clothes changed promptly when problems such as incontinence occur. These residents should have enough outfits so that clean clothes are always available. Suggest that families provide these residents with clothes made of breathable fabrics (e.g., cotton) that minimize smells of perspiration or other odors and are easy to clean. Helping residents who can no longer monitor their own hygiene to stay clean and meet social norms can preserve their dignity and self-esteem.

WHAT THE ENVIRONMENT CAN DO

The presence of unpleasant smells in the environment often negatively affects the mood of residents, staff, and families. Bad smells can make residents irritable, agitated, and more likely to attempt to leave the unit. In turn, this makes more work for staff, who must constantly respond to this disruptive behavior. Unpleasant odors also can reduce both the length and number of visits from families and volunteers. For these reasons, it is important to figure out ways to minimize these odors as much as possible. (See Volume 2, Chapter 4 for a detailed discussion about how to reduce incontinence rates by using environmental, medical, and behavioral approaches.)

Reducing Negative Odors

The key factor in reducing negative odors in the environment is to select materials and finishes that are easy to clean. "Cleanability" must be balanced with visual and tactile interest. Concentrate on placing easily cleaned materials where they are needed most (e.g., use vinyl for seat cushions but fabric on the seat backs).

Odor-resistant carpets are becoming popular in residential facilities; however, these floor coverings must be installed over a sealed surface. Unsealed concrete subfloors are porous and can trap liquids that will leach onto the surface of the carpet no matter how frequently it is cleaned. Nothing can be done about this odor source except to reseal the concrete slab. If the facility is installing or replacing carpet, then the surface of the concrete subfloor should be sealed to ensure that the carpet will perform as expected. Floor sealers are available that have few airborne irritants and can be used while residents are still in the area (ask a carpet installer or sales representative for information). With any new construction, the architect should specify that a floor sealer be applied to the slab after the concrete has set.

Maintenance of cleanable items is equally important. Make sure that there are good policies in place for regular maintenance and spot maintenance. All health care staff members should be responsible for cleaning simple spills or pointing out spots to maintenance and housekeeping staff. Also, review the chemicals that are used to clean and their associated odors. Cleaning chemicals with a less offensive odor or products that are odor-free should be selected.

Do not underestimate the power of fresh air in an indoor environment. One way for facilities to control rising energy costs is for the building systems to frequently circulate the same stale air. If odors are a problem, then the heating/cooling/ventilating system should be reviewed to verify that it is providing a reasonable amount of fresh air. Whenever possible, a window should be opened to allow fresh air into the environment. A locking mechanism that controls the size of the window opening can be used for safety purposes.

Using Positive Smells and Tastes as Room Cues

Introducing positive smells and tastes can help cue residents as to the purpose of certain rooms. For example, the aroma of freshly baked bread or coffee brewing in the dining room will cue residents to mealtimes. The smell of soap or other bath products signals the resident that the activity is bathing in the tub room. A favorite smell such as a lavender sachet on the bedroom door may help a resident with low vision to correctly identify his or her bedroom door.

Using Aromatherapy

Aromatherapy, a technique that introduces pleasant scents into the environment, is gaining popularity among those who care for residents with dementia. Preliminary research indicates that people may respond positively to aromas even when they do not consciously detect them in the environment. Thus, aromatherapy may improve psychological well-being and alertness in residents with dementia. It also gives staff another way to communicate, even with residents with late-stage dementia.

Originally, aromatherapy was used by healers who extracted essential oils from plants, flowers, and trees for their various therapeutic properties. However, specialized knowledge is not necessary to produce a simpler version of aromatherapy in the facility's environment. You can use pleasantly scented lotions, baby powder, fragrant bubble baths, and a variety of pleasing scents to provide positive stimulation for residents. Soothing aromatic oils, such as lavender or sandalwood, can be applied to a lightbulb. When the bulb is turned on, the heat diffuses the aroma throughout the room (see Figure 4.1).

Planting Therapeutic Gardens

Planting special therapeutic gardens is another way to give residents who may not see or hear well rich sensory experiences while outdoors. Different fragrances—the sweet perfume of a rose garden or the various scents in an

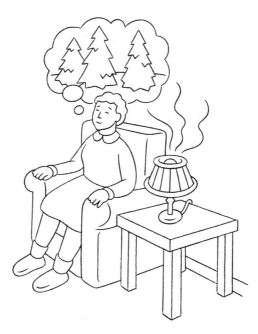

Figure 4.1. Aromatherapy introduces pleasant scents into the environment and is gaining popularity.

herb garden, such as lavender, rosemary, sage, and thyme—can have powerful emotional impact. Choose plants that are fragrant but nontoxic (see Volume 4, Appendix C for a list of nontoxic plants). Therapeutic gardens also
may include items that are interesting for residents to taste, such as mint, pars-
ley, or ripe tomatoes.

♦ ♦ ♦

A summary sheet follows, which condenses the chapter text into a
quick overview. The authors have also provided an area for you to make your
own notes about your own staff and facility. Managerial staff may wish to use
the summary sheets as handouts to accompany direct care staff training, or to
post them by the time clock or nurses' station or include them in staff's pay
envelopes.

SMELL AND TASTE SUMMARY SHEET

1. The sense of smell is linked to the part of the brain that deals with memory processing and emotions. Smells can evoke powerful memories and emotional experiences.
2. The experience of smell may be different in people with Alzheimer's disease.
3. The number of taste buds decreases after age 50, affecting people's experience of taste. Sweet, sour, bitter, and salty discrimination is reduced and enjoyment of food is affected.

What Staff Can Do

1. Incorporate familiar, comforting smells in the facility's environment. Opening a window after the lawn has been mowed, baking cookies in or near the living area, and picking fresh herbs or flowers in the garden may all awaken warm memories.
2. Find out which scents individual residents have enjoyed during their lives and use them in bath or personal care products. Also ask about scents that were disliked or are upsetting. Preferences can be highly personal, and scents can trigger upsetting memories as well as happy ones. Record personal likes and dislikes.
3. Minimize unpleasant odors in the environment by using cleaning products with pleasant and familiar scents, assisting residents with personal hygiene, and keeping the environment clean.
4. The flavor of foods may need to be enhanced for it to be enjoyed. Try making lemonade sweeter and coffee a bit stronger.

What the Environment Can Do

1. When designing the environment, select surfaces that are easy to clean; make sure the concrete subfloor below the carpeting is sealed, and choose carpeting that resists odors.
2. Eliminate negative odors by cleaning problem areas immediately, and incorporate fresh air in the environment.
3. Use familiar smells to cue times of day such as mealtimes and bathtimes, and use each resident's personal favorite scents to help the person find his or her room.
4. Pleasant aromas can support relaxation, alertness, and well-being. For example, fragrant flowering plants and flower garden fragrances can be extremely effective.

YOUR NOTES

5

Touch

Holding someone's hand, patting his or her shoulder, or giving a hug can be therapeutic for residents, who often feel lonely in a nursing facility. These simple gestures show caring and remind older people of being in comfortable family settings.

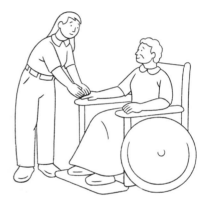

HOW TOUCH CHANGES WITH AGE

The skin is the main organ that conveys tactile sensations to the brain. The skin has a number of other important functions, including acting as a barrier against foreign substances and disease and regulating temperature. With advancing age, some significant changes in the skin normally occur. In general, the epidermis (top layer of skin) loses cells, causing the skin to become drier and less elastic. The dermis (second layer of skin) also deteriorates. As a consequence, the skin loses its resilience and may look like tissue paper that has been crumpled and ironed flat. Because older skin is often fragile, staff always should pat rather than rub it when providing personal care.

A person's sense of touch also tends to decline with aging. Sometimes older people may not sense temperature changes or pain, which can be dangerous for them. Older people are prone to skin damage, including bruises, pressure sores, and cuts. For instance, residents may not notice the pressure on their skin from lying or sitting in the same position too long and may develop sores. Staff should encourage residents to, if possible, get up or change position frequently and check that they are not developing sores on their skin.

There are both physiological and psychological benefits associated with therapeutic touch. The benefits of massage on the nervous, muscular, and circulatory systems can be significant. It also can calm breathing and decrease stress. Hand, foot, back, and shoulder massage help to comfort people in chronic pain or psychological distress. Some related psychological benefits of therapeutic touch include an increased state of relaxation, pleasurable feelings, decreased anxiety, and help with sleep (Stevensen, 1994).

WHAT STAFF CAN DO

Although many kinds of sophisticated technology are used in long-term care, a trend is forming to use simple comforting techniques to improve residents' quality of life. Massage and other forms of healing touch are becoming increasingly popular because long-term care staff can learn them relatively quickly and easily.

Incorporating Touch into Therapeutic Activities

Touch can be used for reminiscence when activities conjure memories of the residents' everyday lives and routines from home. Certain familiar tactile activities such as folding laundry, kneading dough, potting plants, and petting a dog or cat may stimulate residents' memories. Residents at different stages of dementia can still participate in activities involving sensory stimulation. For example, someone who can no longer bake may be able to mix up dough or form it into balls for cookies.

As residents become less mobile, they are not as likely to find interesting sources of tactile stimulation on their own. In too many nursing facilities, low-functioning residents with dementia are starved for sensory stimulation and exhibit behaviors such as rubbing their hands on a tray table or tapping their fingers repeatedly on a hard surface. These residents are showing staff that they need something interesting to hold onto and touch. Offering them objects with interesting textures (e.g., a fur muff, a silk scarf) to handle can substitute for some repetitive behaviors and may be therapeutic.

As residents' fine motor control diminishes, it is necessary to provide larger objects that are easier to handle (Calkins, 1988). Ask families about residents' preferences and provide objects that they like to touch. A former handyman might enjoy a bucket of nuts and bolts and parts, whereas a seamstress may like a basket of interesting fabrics or a collection of large buttons. Some residents may enjoy having something soft to hold, such as a pillow. The

Spinoza Company makes a stuffed bear that, when squeezed, plays prerecorded messages. As with a tape recorder, messages can be recorded by a family member and played back to the resident to offer reassurance and comfort.

There is heated debate regarding whether it is infantilizing for residents with dementia to be given dolls and stuffed animals to hold. The answer to the question of what objects are appropriate for older residents with dementia greatly depends on the personalities and social histories of individual residents. In general, objects that are not childlike are best; however, there are exceptions. If an older woman was formerly a nanny, then she may enjoy caring for and nurturing a doll. Similarly, an animal lover may enjoy cuddling a stuffed animal when a real pet is not available.

Pet therapy is also becoming popular in many nursing facilities. Petting a cat, dog, or rabbit can be relaxing for some older people. Some residents have never lived without a pet. Petting an animal provides tactile stimulation and is a way of communicating that does not require a verbal language. The kind of nonverbal acceptance provided by animals can be positive for residents with dementia who have lost language skills. The Eden Alternative philosophy recommends that, on admission, every resident be given a bird for his or her room (Thomas, 1996). Animals offer unconditional love, which can put a smile on the face of even the saddest resident or one with a severe impairment.

When Touch Is Not Appropriate

In most cases, providing "hands-on" care is greatly appreciated by residents and their family members. Yet, some people do not like to be touched by anyone except their most intimate family members; this should be noted on the personal history sections of their charts. Reasons for these residents' reactions may not be related to their dementia (e.g., a resident who had an abusive husband may prefer to be touched only by female staff members). Documenting these psychosocial factors, pairing residents with appropriate staff, and explaining what will occur during personal care before starting it is likely to minimize combative behavior. At first, staff should approach these residents slowly and touch them gently on a limb, such as their arm. They should not continue to touch them if the touch produces a negative reaction; instead, when possible, they should come back later and try again. This type of individualized care improves the quality of life of the residents and can result in significant savings in staff time by minimizing the likelihood of catastrophic reactions.

WHAT THE ENVIRONMENT CAN DO

Improving the Textural Environment

Texture provides an important form of sensory stimulation for understanding the environment. It can be especially critical for residents with low vision, for whom texture is an important cue that signals surface changes and transitions. Multiple textures also make the environment more visually attractive and provide residents with opportunities to touch different types of surfaces.

Texture that reminds residents of being at home can be added in many ways. Most institutional environments are filled with hard, sterile surfaces. People's houses usually are filled with softer items such as pillows, rugs, and cushions. It is not expensive to add some of these simple touches on the unit. Pillows of different shapes, sizes, and textures can be used throughout a unit if they have removable covers that can be taken off and easily laundered. Upholstery, drapes, and wall hangings also add interesting elements that residents can touch. If these elements are thematic, then they also can serve as orientation cues to help residents more easily locate the wing on which they live (e.g., floral pillows used in the garden wing).

Residents and family members should be encouraged to bring familiar knickknacks and other items from home that residents like to handle. Being surrounded by these familiar items helps them to be more comfortable in the long-term care environment and helps with preserving their sense of self. Some residents may enjoy feeling productive by spending time dusting and arranging the favorite items that they have brought from home. Residents may have an easier time handling larger items with simple parts that can be manipulated.

Contrasting textures in the environment enable residents who do not like to be touched by other people to experience tactile stimulation. For example, residents who resist bathing may come to enjoy this experience if pleasant elements, such as soft terry cloth robes and a towel warmer, are added to the tub room. Some residents may enjoy handling bath accessories and bathing themselves using a soft washcloth or large, brightly colored soft sponge.

Avoiding Abrasive Elements

As skin loses its elasticity, residents are more susceptible to tearing their skin. The facility should avoid purchasing items with sharp corners or abrasive textures. For example, dining tables should have slightly rounded edges so that residents do not rest their arms against a sharp edge (see Volume 2 for more information on furniture choices and options). Wicker-type furniture is popular in long-term care facilities, but it can have an abrasive texture that can feel uncomfortable. In addition, it can deteriorate as it ages. Before purchasing wicker furniture, review the weave of the piece for a relatively smooth surface, and afterward inspect it periodically for wear. The majority of wicker surfaces should be covered with pillows for adequate support and more comfortable seating. Carefully inspect the arms of wicker furniture to see whether they provide a smooth surface and good support when rising. Avoid using wicker dining tables, which can be uncomfortable to lean arms against. Glass tops on wicker tables also can be difficult to rest against and can be a hazard for residents whose balance is unstable.

Regulating Temperature

Residents with reduced touch sensitivity may not respond quickly to dangerous conditions. Although water temperature frequently is regulated by the states, the facility always should make sure that its hot water will not scald residents. Antiscald devices should be installed at all plumbing fixtures where residents may be at risk. Older people also are affected by drafts and changes in air temperature. Keep residents' temperature preferences in mind when adjusting thermostats and airflow.

◆ ◆ ◆

A summary sheet follows, which condenses the chapter text into a quick overview. The authors have also provided an area for you to make your own notes about your own staff and facility. Managerial staff may wish to use the summary sheets as handouts to accompany direct care staff training, or to post them by the time clock or nurses' station or include them in staff's pay envelopes.

THE SENSES SUMMARY SHEET

1. Touch is an important part of the human experience. Holding a hand or getting or giving a hug can be therapeutic. The skin is the main organ that conveys tactile information to the brain.

2. With age, the top layer of the skin becomes dry and loses elasticity. As the layers below deteriorate, resilience declines and skin may become quite fragile.

3. The sense of touch also declines and residents may be less aware of possible injury to the skin or of extreme temperatures.

What Staff Can Do

1. Carefully document individual residents' comfort levels with being touched. Although touch is an important part of the human experience, people vary in their comfort levels. A touch on the hand, a pat on the back, or a hug can be comforting or discomforting, depending on the resident and the relationship to the person touching him or her. Remember that assistance with personal care tasks may be difficult if an individual has a low threshold for touch.

2. Provide massage and other forms of healing touch that may be comforting to residents.

3. Incorporate tactile experiences such as kneading dough, folding different fabrics, petting animals, and sorting nuts and bolts or buttons into activity programs.

4. Note unusual behaviors in residents, such as persistently rubbing a table or tapping fingers on a hard surface or along a wall, which may indicate that they need more stimulation, especially tactile stimulation.

5. Include pets in the living environment. This therapeutic intervention is an increasingly popular way to provide residents with tactile stimulation as well as with unconditional love.

What the Environment Can Do

1. Provide residents with tactile cues such as different floor textures or wall textures that signal a transition to another room or area. Multiple textures also make living spaces more interesting and stimulating. Texture can be provided with objects such as throw pillows, draperies, and wall hangings.

2. Provide familiar items (e.g., warm, soft towels) and knickknacks from residents' homes also add texture to the living environment and invite comforting touch.

3. Use textures to encourage residents' comfort during assistance with ADLs.

4. Prevent skin tears by avoiding the installation of abrasive or sharp surfaces, such as tables or counters with sharp corners.

5. Monitor water temperature for residents who have reduced tactile sensitivity.

6. Avoid drafts and abrupt changes in air temperature in the living environment.

YOUR NOTES

Bibliography

American Society of Heating, Refrigerating and Air-Conditioning Engineers, Inc. (1999). *Energy standard for buildings except low-rise residential buildings* (ASHRAE/IESNA Standard 90.1-1999). Atlanta: Author.

Baucom, A.H. (1996). *Hospitality design for the graying generation: Meeting the needs of a growing market.* New York: John Wiley & Sons.

Bowlby, C. (1993). *Therapeutic activities with persons disabled by Alzheimer's disease and related disorders.* Gaithersburg, MD: Aspen Publishers.

Brawley, E.C. (1997). *Designing for Alzheimer's disease: Strategies for creating better environments.* New York: John Wiley & Sons.

Calkins, M.P. (1988). *Design for dementia: Planning environments for the elderly and the confused.* Owings Mills, MD: National Health Publishing.

Calkins, M.P. (1996). *Conceptualizing and assessing environmental press in special care units for people with dementia.* Doctoral dissertation, School of Architecture and Urban Planning, University of Wisconsin–Milwaukee.

Evans, L.K. (1991). Nursing care and management of behavioral problems in the elderly. In M.S. Harper (Ed.), *Management and care of the elderly: Psychosocial perspectives* (pp. 191–206). Newbury Park, CA: Sage Publications.

Hall, G., & Buckwalter, K. (1987). Progressively lowered stress threshold: A conceptual model for care of adults with Alzheimer's disease. *Archives of Psychiatric Nursing, 1*(6), 399–406.

Illuminating Engineering Society of North America. (1998). *Lighting and the visual environment for senior living* (RP-28-98). New York: IESNA.

Kearney, D. (1992). *The new ADA: Compliance and costs.* Kingston, MA: R.S. Means Co.

Lawton, M.P., & Nahemow, L. (1973). Ecology and the aging process. In C. Eisdorfer & M.P. Lawton (Eds.), *Psychology of adult development and aging* (pp. 619–674). Washington, DC: American Psychological Association.

McGuinness, W.J., Stein, B., & Reynolds, J.S. (1980). *Mechanical and electrical equipment for buildings.* New York: John Wiley & Sons.

Nissenboim, S., & Vroman, C. (1998). *The positive interactions program of activities for people with Alzheimer's disease.* Baltimore: Health Professions Press.

Stevensen, C.J. (1994). The psychophysiological effects of aromatherapy massage following cardiac surgery. *Complementary Therapies in Medicine, 2,* 27–35.

Thomas, W. (1996). *Life worth living. How someone you love can still enjoy life in a nursing home: The Eden Alternative in action.* Acton, MA: VanderWyk & Burnham.

Tideiksaar, R. (1997). *Falling in old age: Prevention and management* (2nd ed.). New York: Springer Publishing.

Witucki, J., & Twibell, R. (1997). The effect of sensory stimulation activities on the psychological well being of patients with advanced Alzheimer's disease. *American Journal of Alzheimer's Disease, 12*(1), 10–15.

Index

Page numbers followed by *f* indicate figures; those followed by *t* indicate tables. This is a comprehensive index covering Volumes 1–4 of *Creating Successful Dementia Care Settings*. The first number of each entry indicates the volume; the second number indicates the page.

creating areas for, 3.68–3.69, 3.70, 3.72
  rummaging drawers, 3.29, 3.70
  sensory stimulation boards, 3.71
  "workplaces," 3.71
  environmental adjustments for, 3.74
  and interfering with others, 3.70
  redirecting, 4.84
  needing to feel productive and,
    3.66–3.67, 3.69
  and privacy, 4.80
  stimulation, increasing, 3.69
  triggers, 3.65
  and wandering, 3.10
  see also Hoarding

Safe Return, 3.45, 3.58
Safety, and residents with dementia,
    2.50–2.53
Scolding, ineffectiveness of, 3.114
Sensory cues, see Hearing; Smell (sense
    of); Taste, age-related changes in;
    Touch; Vision
Sensory impairments, 1.1
  and cognitive impairment, 1.2
  and mobility, 2.45
Sensory Stimulation Assessment form,
    3.133–3.134
  use of, 3.48, 3.92, 3.131–3.132
Sensory stimuli, 1.1
  and activities for people with
    dementia, 1.3
  conflicting, 1.3–1.4
  and hallucinations, 1.3
  impact on people with dementia,
    1.2–1.3
  quality of, 1.3
  tactile stimulation, importance of,
    3.66, 3.67f, 3.113
    special napkins, 3.72
Sequencing cards, 2.94, 2.100, 3.86
  dressing, 2.153–2.154, 2.162
Sexual advances, 3.119
Sexual behaviors, residents'
  between residents, 3.116–3.117
  between residents and nonresidents,
    3.115–3.116
  facility policies, 3.114–3.115
  inappropriate, 3.107–3.110, 3.117–3.120
  staff training, 3.115, 3.121, 3.122
  see also Consent, informed
Sexually ambiguous behavior, 3.110

Shadow boxes, 2.40, 3.25, 3.33
Shadowing, 3.40
Shelving, 4.22–4.23, 4.23f, 4.162, 4.162f
Shoes
  dressing, 2.155
  effective for mobility, 2.69–2.70
Showering, 2.175
  shower curtains, half height, 2.175,
    2.179, 3.89, 3.99
  shower manufacturers, 2.178–2.179
  shower wands, hand-held, 2.175, 3.88,
    3.89f
  see also Bathing
Side-entry bathtub with door, see
    Bathtubs
Side-entry tilting bathtub, see Bathtubs
Signage
  appropriate, 2.39–2.40, 3.32–3.33,
    3.60–3.61
    as detour cue, 3.28
    directional, 2.25f, 2.34f, 2.100
    and hazardous areas, 3.28
    and lighting, 2.26
    placement, 2.27–2.28
    as reorientation device, 3.25
  inappropriate, 2.27f
Single-tipped cane, 2.64t
Skin care, 1.41
Slide transfer benches, 2.175, 2.179
Smell (sense of)
  age-related changes in, 1.33
    environmental adjustments for, 1.39
  aromatherapy, 1.37
  food as a sensory cue, 1.37
  and personal care, see Personal care,
    providing
Socially inappropriate behaviors,
    3.105–3.122
Spa model of care, see Hospitality model
    of care
Spatial adjacencies, 2.18–2.19
  cluster floor plan, 2.23–2.24
  double-loaded corridors, 2.19–2.21,
    2.19f, 2.20f
  pavilion floor plan, 2.21–2.23
  and residential character in long-term
    care facilities, 4.116–4.118, 4.118f,
    4.119f
Staffing patterns, 2.54–2.55
Stimulation
  limiting, 3.48
  providing, 3.45–3.46, 3.46f

Wandering, 3.1, 3.9–3.11, 3.10*t*,
  3.36–3.37
  activity programming, 3.29–3.31, 3.36
  and agenda behavior, 3.4
  and agenda behavior approach,
    3.14–3.15, 3.15*f*
  and disorientation, 3.16
    cues to reorientation, 3.20
  environmental adjustments for,
    3.21–3.29
  excessive walking, *see* Excessive walking
  and furniture as intervention,
    3.21–3.22, 3.22*f*, 4.86
  limiting, 3.28–3.29
  monitoring systems, 3.29, 3.33–3.34,
    3.56, 3.61–3.62
  motivators for, 3.11, 3.12*t*
  and nonwanderers, differences
    between, 3.11
  perceptions about, 3.21
  and programming, 3.15–3.16
    engaging previous interests,
      3.16–3.18
    structured activities, 3.18–3.19
  and reality orientation, 3.19–3.20
  and redirection, 3.13–3.14, 3.14*f*,
    3.36
  and resident's anxiety, 3.16
  and restraints, 3.12
Water, and bathing, 2.172, 2.175; *see also*
  Bathing

Wayfinding, and orientation, 2.11–2.12,
  2.13
  dementia and, 2.14, 2.16, 2.18; *see also*
    Color; Signage; Spatial
    adjacencies
  see also specific rooms
Wealshire, The, 4.117–4.118, 4.119*f*
Well-being, feelings of, 4.95–4.97
Wheelchairs, 2.65
Windows
  and excess noise, treatments for, 1.29
  and exiting residents, 3.58
  and glare, 1.18, 2.74
    blinds, 1.18–1.19, 3.95
    reducing, to prevent combative
      behaviors, 3.95–3.97
  treatments, bedroom, 4.28–4.29
  and ventilation, residents' control
    over, 4.103
Withdrawal, social
  and diminishment of functional
    abilities, 2.1–2.2
    dementia, 2.7
    mobility problems, 2.44
    orientation problems, 2.13
  and low vision, 1.10
  and threats to privacy needs, 4.79
Work life roles, and activities planning,
  4.53
  creating workplaces, 4.60
  workshops, 4.61–4.62, 4.61*f*

ORDER THESE COMPANION VIDEOS FOR CREATING SUCCESSFUL DEMENTIA CARE SETTINGS

Video 1
Maximizing Cognitive and Functional Abilities/No. 2769/40-min VHS/$92

Video 2
Minimizing Disruptive Behaviors/No. 2777/21-min VHS/$55

Video 3
Enhancing Self and Sense of Home/No. 2785/33-min VHS/$78

Prices are subject to change.

ORDER FORM

Please send me the following video(s):

Stk No.	Title	Quantity	Price

	Subtotal	
	MD residents, add 5% tax	
	Shipping & Handling	
	TOTAL	

SHIPPING & HANDLING

For pre-tax total of	Add
$0.00 to $49.99	$5.00
$50.00 to $399.99	10%
$400.00 and over	8%

❏ Check enclosed (payable to **Health Professions Press**)
❏ Bill my institution (attach purchase order) ❏ MasterCard ❏ Visa ❏ AmEx

Credit card#/Exp. date _____

Signature _____

Name _____

Address _____
(Orders cannot be shipped to P.O. boxes)

City/State/ZIP _____

Daytime phone _____

HEALTH PROFESSIONS PRESS P.O. BOX 10624 BALTIMORE, MD 21285-0624
TOLL FREE (888) 337-8808 FAX (410) 337-8539
www.healthpropress.com

ZCK